101 TIPS for RECOVERING from TRAUMATIC BRAIN INJURY

Practical Advice for TBI Surviors, Caregivers and Teachers

KELLY BOULDIN DARMOFAL

Loving Healing Press

101 Tips for Recovering from Traumatic Brain Injury: Practical Advice for TBI Survivors, Caregivers, and Teachers.
ISBN-13: 978-1-61599-433-5
Copyright © 2015, 2019 by Kelly Bouldin Darmofal

Library of Congress Cataloging-in-Publication Data
Darmofal, Kelly Bouldin, 1977-
101 tips for recovering from traumatic brain injury : practical advice for TBI survivors, caregivers, and teachers / Kelly Bouldin Darmofal ; foreword by Dr. Frank Balch Wood.
      pages cm
Includes bibliographical references.
ISBN 978-1-61599-282-9 (pbk. : alk. paper) -- ISBN 978-1-61599-283-6 (ebook)
1. Brain--Wounds and injuries--Treatment. I. Title. II. Title: One hundred one tips for recovering from traumatic brain injury.
RD594.D37 2015
617.4'81044--dc23
                                  2015028820

Published by
Loving Healing Press
5145 Pontiac Trail
Ann Arbor, MI 48105

Tollfree 888-761-6268 (USA/CAN)
FAX: 734-663-6861
info@LHPress.com
www.LHPress.com

Distributed by Ingram (USA/CAN), New Leaf (USA), and Bertram's Books (UK/EU)

Contents

Foreword

Kelly Bouldin Darmofal's account is unique, yet widely applicable: she teaches any who have suffered TBI—and all who love, care for, and teach them—insights that are not only novel but revolutionary...

Like Job, she learned the hard lesson of a faith that ultimately made her both "thankful to my non-intervening God," as she put it, and for that reason, resolute in becoming the person she now is. Her experiences exemplify that providence can't be preached—to self or others—apart from persistent self-actualization.

Warnings against inflexible educational bureaucracy abound in her descriptions of narrow-minded teaching. Yet, she recognizes good teaching so well that she becomes a teacher herself and models what all teachers must emulate: respect for students as persons in all their idiosyncratic potential. She understands mediocrity as the great millstone around the neck of education.

The book is not simply worth reading; it is necessary reading for patients, poets, professors, preachers, and teachers.

Dr. Frank Balch Wood

(Frank Wood is professor emeritus of neurology-neuropsychology at Wake Forest School of Medicine and an ordained Baptist minister.)

Introduction

The following "tips" were compiled by TBI survivor, Kelly Bouldin Darmofal, whose memoir *Lost in My Mind: Recovering from TBI* was published in 2014 by Modern History Press. Some insights come from her mother/primary caretaker, Carolyn Bouldin, a teacher who choreographed Kelly's reentry into public high school. Both Kelly and Carolyn experienced first-hand the perils and hardships experienced post-TBI by millions of Americans; TBI is a "silent illness," many say, and the symptoms include long and short term memory loss, the inability to think and speak rapidly, the loss of muscle control, and other impairments that vary according to the severity of the TBI. Their life strategies may or may not apply to all TBI survivors, but they exemplify probable issues those with TBI may confront. Kelly's main advice is "Never give up!"

Tips For TBI Survivors

1. REALIZE YOU ARE NOT ALONE because in America there are at least 2.5 million new cases of TBI yearly.

2. Let your fears motivate you to NEVER GIVE UP… face what you fear, one obstacle at a time.

3. DENIAL can both *hurt and help* you; however, you must learn to accept your body's recovery pace.

4. SMILE at those who think they understand TBI while encouraging you to accept less than you desire from life.

5. ASSUME NOTHING – the disabilities of each TBI survivor are unique, yet similarities do exist. You will need to discover for yourself if you recall basic skills, such as matching shoes and clothing or reading and writing from left to right.

6. KNOW THE DIFFERENCE BETWEEN LOW IQ AND RETROGRADE AMNESIA - Not knowing basic things doesn't indicate low IQ...it may indicate retrograde amnesia, or long-term memory loss.

7. DEVISE UNIQUE WAYS TO RELEARN FORGOTTEN SKILLS -

    For example, you could sing rap lyrics to improve slow speech patterns.

8. SEPARATE YOUR WARDROBE INTO OUTFITS THAT YOU CAN SEE - Things in the back of the closet may be forgotten. For the TBI survivor, if you can't see it, it may not exist!

9. KEEP LISTS, USE POST-ITS...short term memory loss is common after a TBI...it's OK to write on your arm because anterograde amnesia can make you crazy, especially when you can't locate the keys you just tossed somewhere.

10. WRITE DOWN EVERYTHING...to alleviate future frustrations, record information you want to remember or are scared you might forget.

11. STAY ORGANIZED – keep things in one place and visible if possible so you won't forget where they are.

12. TRY NOT TO ARGUE WITH PEOPLE. An argument may or may not be socially inappropriate behavior, so use the ambiguous response, *"You may be right!"*

13. If you know you are prone to socially inappropriate language, PRACTICE TALKING TO STRANGERS who won't get upset; you might go out of town to practice skills that once were basic, and avoid embarrassing friends and family.

14. USE BIG WORDS for a dual purpose: "azure" may be easier to recall than "blue," and people think you are still smart if you raise your vocabulary, or utilize proper diction when conversing.

15. USE "PARDON ME?" INSTEAD OF "WHAT?" You may find people talk too fast at first, and you need to ask them to repeat things. Receptive and expressive processing disorders are common following head injury. If you say "What? What?" people think you aren't listening …if you say "Pardon?" they assume intelligence.

16. THE OLD YOU is someone people say they miss, when there is only one you; simply nod your head and tell them that "trauma changes a person." You can also blame any bad habits on the "old you."

17. MEMORIZE NEW DATA BY SETTING THINGS TO MUSIC OR RHYME.

    ("Amendment One is easy to teach…freedom of Religion and Press and Speech!")

18. RELY ON COMPUTERS…they are your friends and don't criticize. Devices like iPhones and iPads have apps designed to help you remember things.

19. REACH OUT TO FRIENDS AND TELL THEM IF YOU NEED HELP…*they don't read minds.*

20. WEAR BLACK…then everything matches!!

21. DON'T INVEST IN EXPENSIVE CLOTHES OR SUNGLASSES…you may forget where you put them; don't get upset over losing "stuff." Remember – most things can be replaced.

22. LEARN THE FINE ART OF GROVELING: Example for students: teachers like you better if you make eye contact and sit up front.

23. To improve RETROGRADE AMNESIA (long term memory loss), watch historical films to help recall history—movies reinforce memory. Purchase a globe to remind yourself of where things happen(ed). Watch your own home movies, too, to recall how you felt about family and friends – explore your own personality.

24. Expect problems each day, and make a list of how many repetitions it takes for you to relearn/regain a small skill. By RECORDING REPETITIONS, you'll see yourself improve.

25. When cooking or using appliances (as heating pads), make sure electronic devices are turned off before leaving the room – AUTOMATIC SHUT-OFFS can help greatly as well!

26. Place CLOCKS IN EVERY ROOM in the house, to help you stay on schedule.

27. Use stopwatches or timers when cooking to prevent memory difficulties in the kitchen... TIMERS ATTACHED TO CORDS that you can wear around your neck are the most effective. If you leave the kitchen, the alarm will still sound and notify you to return to your cooking.

28. Keep regularly used OBJECTS (keys, glasses) IN ONE frequently visited and visible AREA.

29. Look yourself over in a full-length MIRROR prior to leaving the house to make sure your clothing and accessories match; this also helps you recall things to bring home!

30. READ THE LAWS REGARDING DISABIL-ITY (IDEA for school / Individuals with Disabilities Education Act)...and the ADA (Americans with Disabilities Act) for work. *The law usually favors the handicapped.* (See #31)

31. WHEN YOU ARE ABLE, ADVOCATE FOR YOURSELF! Students should take copies of medical records, IEP, etc. to each teacher every year; don't rely on guidance too much. If you are older and working, provide employers with a letter stating you are disabled (and a list of TBI-related symptoms); that's all you owe an employer – you are probably protected from losing a job you can accomplish by the Americans with Disabilities Act.

32. USE SOCIAL MEDIA for support (*imlostinmymind.com*, that's me!).

33. PARTNER UP: Ask a parent or caretaker to read along with you; ask the schools for *double books*; then you can discuss data you may forget as you read. At work, ally with a mentor.

34. YOU CAN STILL WORK at something meaningful even during recovery. Volunteer at an animal shelter, wash cars, or answer phones at a help desk!

35. FRIENDS IN LOW PLACES may be better than friends in high places.

36. DON'T GIVE IN TO DESPAIR; you are a role model for other survivors, and things do get better!

37. FIND A GOOD PSYCHIATRIST or other counselor as soon as possible, the best you can afford.

38. MAKE SOMEONE ELSE HAPPY each day... especially on days you cannot be happy yourself.

39. RESCUE A PET (I prefer doggie love, but cats may work as well).

40. Tell hairdressers, doctors, etc., NOT TO CHARGE you when (not if) you forget an appointment because you have a traumatic brain injury!

41.   DON'T GRIEVE over friends who forget you; look around for the wonderful new friends who will embrace you.

42.   Give yourself LIMITED TIME TO GRIEVE for lost friends or abilities. When that time is over, put the negative feelings away. (A short "pity party" is OK.)

43.   KEEP A JOURNAL of anything you find useful, from a "no chop" recipe if your hands tremble, to a list of occupations you can one day imagine yourself performing.

44.   LOVE IS POSSIBLE even if you don't have it yet – everyone has idiosyncrasies.

45.   DO NOT FEEL GUILTY ABOUT YOUR TBI; guilt is the only non-productive emotion ("regret" is OK).

46.   Drive a car with MULTIPLE AIRBAGS – when you *can* drive – and LANDMARK LOCATIONS to prevent getting lost (or use a GPS).

47.   Doctors are not omniscient; they cannot know how hard you will work. ONLY YOU CAN KNOW how far you're willing to go to regain what you've lost.

48.   If possible, FIND AN ATTORNEY to handle insurance issues in an affordable way.

49. Listen to yourself on TAPE, and watch yourself on VIDEO – even if it's scary and depressing. You have to know what you're up against. (Use this to support you on tip #50.)

50. Compare your writing, your voice, etc., from month to month—DON'T RELY ON OTHERS to honestly note your improvements.

51. VISIT FORMER CARETAKERS, from nurses to therapists; show them what they meant to your recovery. They may even discover improvements you have missed or forgotten.

52. PICK UP THAT PHONE! Some people are scared to call you and they really do want to stay in touch and help. If you have slow or slurred speech, you can always text people you want to contact.

53. SHARE any "tip" that you find helpful; it may be the one thing another survivor needs to know (I use 3 alarm clocks to awaken every morning).

54. READ – if you can only follow a brief poem, read that; expand to short stories with two characters and advance over time to longer works.

55.   HELP OTHER VICTIMS – write local colleges or universities to demand classes to train teachers of those with TBI; correspond with other survivors; join a support group if you enjoy this; write your Congressman for better legislation regarding TBI survivors.

56.   One visit to an attorney specializing in EMPLOYMENT ISSUES may be worth the fee!

57.   EXPECT LITTLE FAILURES because you want to speed up the healing process, which may have to progress slowly.

58.   Try to remember that YOU'RE NOT THE ONLY PERSON with health issues; *find your lost empathy for others.* Volunteer to help someone else with disabilities; a few hours a week or month will pay back in huge dividends to your self-esteem.

59.   FATIGUE IS NORMAL. Rest when you can! As you sleep, your brain continues to heal.

60.   LAUGH as much as possible and LEARN SOMETHING NEW EVERY DAY! Acquiring new knowledge helps the brain form new neural connections.

Tips for Friends and Caregivers

61. TELL THE TRUTH- HONESTY helps the healing process. If friends exaggerate and say, "You look super," the victim of TBI knows the truth. Rather, say, "You did better today than yesterday…but we'll get there together!"

62. GIVE HOPE – friends can express optimism or pessimism. Those who truly help will, in small ways, show they expect the victim of TBI to get fully well.

    NO ONE CAN DO ANYTHING THEY DON'T BELIEVE THEY CAN DO!

63. Help THE VICTIM OF TBI FIGURE OUT WHAT THEY REMEMBER AND WHAT THEY DO NOT.

64. FILL IN LOSTS MEMORIES with photographs, videos, and conversations. You might have some photos on your Facebook timeline that may help jog memory.

65. STAY POSITIVE AND OPTIMISTIC; pessimism is a luxury no one can afford.

66. USE SIMILIES AND METAPHORS IN YOUR SPEECH to help TBI survivors transit from a literal world to the figurative; "I'm angry as a football coach," is better than "I'm mad."

67. EXPLAIN words with multiple meanings: Note the difference between a "hot" day and a "hot" girl.

68. PREPARE FOR MULTIPLE REPETITIONS because new knowledge is more difficult for TBI survivors to retain than old knowledge.

69. Take the time to SHARE YOUR UNIQUE GIFTS, interests, and hobbies. Take your loved one with TBI to your baseball game, a movie...new survivors can't perform well yet, and need to be entertained and to enjoy life.

70. TIME is key; take the time to allow survivors to FEEL NEEDED...actively do charitable things for others.

71. DESPAIR IS NOT AN OPTION – sing, laugh, and move forward hour by hour.

72. Gather your own support network as CARETAKERS NEED THEIR OWN CARE-TAKERS; ask for help when life changes instantaneously.

73. Keep a LIST BY THE TELEPHONE of current events (sports events, movie reviews) to give survivors topics to talk about when they are in a mental flood of confusion.

74. Plan "SAFE OUTINGS" with trustworthy drivers; make sure they (and you) have a rider on their automobile insurance with protection from the under and/or uninsured motorist.

75. Set up FUTURE EVENTS that survivors can plan for – a short cruise, for instance, involves no driving...and the survivors are less likely to get lost in a boat on the ocean.

76. Set SHORT-TERM goals – survivors can learn to jump a rope, read and discuss a poem, make a sandwich; long-term goals will follow but are less important immediately following a TBI.

77. PREPARE FOR DIFFICULT QUESTIONS, and answer honestly if asked, "Do people expect sex on a first date? Do I look OK?"

78. Try to ASSESS THE MENTAL AGE level of the survivor; the recovery period may feel like (and actually be) a delayed adolescence.

79. Confront inevitable depression; FIND A THERAPIST/PSYCHIATRIST who can offer

both counseling and medication to caretaker as well as survivor.

80. READ UP ON PTSD (post traumatic stress disorder) so you can confront it at need.

81. Play games like SCRABBLE to enhance spelling skills, or JIGSAW PUZZLES to assist with occupational therapy.

82. Help devise strategies for specific problems; for example, use duct tape to make the OFF position quite easy to find on the eyes of stovetops.

83. If memory issues complicate daily life, have MORE THAN ONE COPY OF IMPOR-TANT ITEMS or documents – spare house and car keys, duplicate drivers' licenses, and so on.

84. USE THE INTERNET to locate information on TBI, from survivor memoirs to legal changes regarding disability law.

85. SOFTWARE can be a recovery miracle: programs to assist with memory, aphasia, and other problems are well worth the investment.

86. Make sure you are not the sole (and weary) caretaker; others have unique skill sets to offer one recovering from TBI, and social

skills may call for a VARIETY OF
COMPANIONS.

87. Help the survivor discover what hobbies are
    still worthwhile and possible; if, for instance,
    skiing is "out," REPLACE THIS HOBBY
    with interesting options (photography,
    writing).

88. Be your loved one's BEST FRIEND, and not
    his/her WORST ENEMY – allow the TBI
    survivor to do whatever she/he can do
    without aid. Independence needs practice and
    not enabling.

89. Consider that LEARNING (memorizing,
    taking tests, reading, writing) is the best
    COGNITIVE THERAPY for those with TBI;
    encourage continuing education at any age
    level.

90. Keep a LIST OF "POSSIBLE FUTURES" you
    observe for your TBI survivor (such as a jury
    clerk, A non-profit coordinator, A teacher?).

91. Keep aiming higher, and DON'T SKIP
    RECOVERY STEPS; the world is changing
    for the better regarding TBI survivors, and a
    handicap can be an advantage in the working
    world.

Tips for Teachers of TBI Survivors

(This section reflects Kelly's belief that going to school was her best cognitive therapy.)

92. Make it a priority to FOLLOW a TBI survivor's IEP – Individual Education Program – at all times. Deviating from this list of modifications will send the student into an immediate FLOOD, or state of panic.

93. Realize that THE STUDENT WITH A RECENT TBI IS HEALING; the person you see will be different next month and possibly tomorrow. Coleridge calls this "a willing suspension of disbelief."

94. MAKE NO ASSUMPTIONS; can this survivor recall the multiplication tables? Read/write from left to right? Explore and set immediate priorities.

95. NEVER CONDESCEND, for this wounded student may be smarter than you, but unable to speak coherently for a time. PRACTICE PATIENCE!

96. Allow LEEWAY FOR THE FAMILY – give home phone numbers/emails of teachers and counselors, and possibly self-selection of teachers.

97. DARE TO SET A PRECEDENT (can physical therapy count as physical education in your school district?).

98. KEEP A SENSE OF HUMOR – for instance if the TBI survivor uses socially inappropriate language – most likely a reminder given with a smile will work best.

99. Use teaching modifications, such as these:

- TRIGGERS to assist with recall: "D" may help the student remember "Dante."
- WORD BANKS for testing (as a list of all states when the answer is "North Carolina").
- NOTETAKERS and ORAL TESTING as needed.
- MNEMONIC STRATEGIES to aid in recall.
- EXTENDED TIME for assignments; give all assignments IN WRITING.
- FREQUENT REST BREAKS; fatigue is a symptom of TBI.

100. NEVER POSTPONE A TEST! Your student may have been up all night memorizing work that will fade in a few hours; generally, the memory capacity of the student with TBI improves over time.

101. DEMAND EDUCATION concerning how to best instruct those with TBI; online courses are available for continuing education, and the BIAA (Brain Injury Association of America) can help. Have you heard of Child Find? Are you prepared to teach diagnostically and recognize symptoms of TBI? BE READY! The TBI population is growing into the millions.

~ ~ ~

The Caretaker
by Carolyn Bouldin

I never danced the dying swan
Or molded forms in clay.
I never penned a single page
One might recall today,
But I have heard the muse
And all the gods of life conspire
And lived as choreographer
Of someone else's fire.

Read: Even if Reading is Nearly Impossible

When I awoke from coma in the fall of 1992, I had no knowledge of traumatic brain injury. I simply wanted to regain my powers of speech, which came slowly over months and years. Yet I had a larger problem: I could not comprehend slang, the complexity of speech, or the nuances of humor. My friends spoke to me, yet their words were ambiguous, and even simple phrases like "Catch you later!" left me confused…why catch me? Did I fall?

Thus I tell you plainly that poetry alone helped me understand the variety of meanings contained within words. I needed brief simple poems to help me reach into my mind for forgotten abilities. "The night has a thousand eyes," wrote Francis William Bourdillon. My own eyes were impaired by TBI, and a teacher read me this poetic line. Suddenly I realized that the "eyes" represented stars, and a whole new world opened up for me. One word could convey many meanings. I read more poems, and asked others to read them to me. I especially liked the work of Langston Hughes, and his recurring motif of dreams. Almost a century ago he wrote: "Hold fast to dreams/ For when dreams go/ Life is a barren field/Frozen with snow." My injured brain was frozen, too, and I needed to dream of a better future.

But I was afraid to return to school in 1993. I still limped and staggered and fell. But I didn't want my life to be a "barren field."

Yet I had to return, said my doctors. In order to remember the myriad things I'd forgotten, I had to immerse myself in the familiar. As Alice Walker writes in her novel *The Temple of My Familiar*, "What you hope for, you also fear." Yet in 1993 I couldn't read an entire novel because I forgot characters and plotlines too quickly. (I read my first novel with comprehension ten years post-TBI). Nevertheless, I returned to high school, and was blessed with wonderful English teachers.

In my sophomore year of high school English, my teacher assigned Plato's "Allegory of the Cave" to our class. *Strangely I remember its message now, when I had huge difficulty remembering it for a test years ago.* In the allegory, a group of people lived far beneath the earth in caves, and never for a moment were aware of the existence of sunlight. One man dared to climb out of his underground cavern, finding himself exulting at last in the light of day. His sublime ecstasy made him wonder how he could have survived in the darkness for so long. Yet this man decided, ultimately, to return to the dark cave below. He felt responsible to those left behind, and felt called to teach them of the light up above.

I believe that it is appropriate to go back into the shadows in order to teach others about the possibility of a better life. Educators do this, and most likely Plato's allegory led me back to the special education classroom.

Today the only reason I can bear to discuss my head injury is in hopes that my experience may give some hope to other victims, hope that they can overcome their infirmities, or at least find some way to compensate for them. Writers communicate despair and hope, sorrow and suffering, but almost always the sense that one is not alone in the world.

Words have become extremely important to me, for I know what it means not to have them, not to use them. Writing can be simple and short like a poem, which is why "101 Tips" is designed in a simple and brief format.

In the *Winston-Salem Journal* (February 19, 2000) friend and former editor John Gates wrote in "The Dumbing of America" that: "In 1950, the average 14-year-old American had a vocabulary of 25,000 words. The latest estimate puts the vocabulary for the average 14-year-old U. S. student at 10,000 words." This is a tragedy beyond belief. While I do believe that verbal expression needs speed more than quality, I also believe that quality is important. It is important to read broadly, expanding from short to longer works.

The first TBI memoir that influenced me was written by Dr. Claudia Osborn. Her autobiographical book *Over My Head: A Doctor's Own Story of Head Injury from the Inside Looking Out* was published in 1998, and my mother read most of it to me. Dr. Osborn wrote in the first person, carefully explaining that many victims of head injury cannot remember certain events or describe them well enough to actually speak in the first person.

She relied on her journals and the journals and memories of others to recall important material. I learned from Dr. Osborn that using my own mother's journals could help me to write my own memoir: *Lost in My Mind: Recovering from Traumatic Brain Injury* (TBI) published in 2014 by Modern History Press. One tip I learned: Dr. Osborn uses an alarm clock in her automobile; it is set to go off every three minutes to remind her to recall where she is going. (She often places her destination in a note within the car.) Is she on her way to lecture first year me student? To the grocery store? Home? She hears a RING... consults, her note, and BINGO! She reaches the right destination. I suffered Claudia Osborn's degree of short-term memory loss only temporarily, but can identify with what it feels like to be very intelligent, and still lack certain memory skills.

Other memoirs became interesting to me because I didn't have to follow a plot. Holocaust survivors can speak to a TBI survivor, because they have overcome impossible odds to regain their humanity and reason. I am especially fond of *Man's Search for Meaning* by Victor Frankl, in which he wrote: "Those who have a 'why' to live, can bear with almost any 'how'." From Frankl I learned to pursue meaning in my life, which is currently to acquaint America's educational system with the needs of students with TBI. In 2016 I will teach a course for education students at Salem College in North Carolina, and hopefully I can spark awareness of the "silent illness" of TBI to help millions of American student survivors.

In 2002 I successfully read and enjoyed a novel – probably because of the format used by author Dean Koontz. *The Watchers* fascinated me as the stories of two separate characters converged slowly, one drawn by circumstance to the other. I could follow two characters as they joined with the help of an unusual dog who could spell out sentences using Scrabble tiles. OK, so Scrabble was one of the tools I used to relearn spelling skills. But *Watchers* enabled me to find a bit of magic in the world of TBI, and led me into the wonderful healing world of canine rescue.

Today in 2015, I still enjoy short fiction and poetry. I can, however, follow other survivor stories such as Laura Hillenbrand's *Unbroken: A World War II Story of Survival, Resilience, and Redemp-*

tion. The world is filled with survivors, and those with TBI are not alone.

For those who prefer brevity I recommend Gary Trudeau's *Signature Wound: Rocking TBI*. The character Toggle has expressive aphasia as I did (and do), yet he pursues his career and his relationships despite adversity.

As to my personal quest to educate teachers about the needs of TBI survivors, I recommend following the website of the Brain Injury Association of America: *www.biausa.org*. I recommend the following study for those interested in TBI and education:

Gordon, W. A., Oswald, J. M., Vaughn, S. L., Connors, S. H., & Brown, M. (2013). State of the states: Meeting the educational needs of children with traumatic brain injury. BIAA.

Also of interest is a study which suggests an inexpensive method of training educators about the needs of TBI survivors which is:

Glang, A., Tyler, J., Pearson, S., Todis, B., & Morvant, M. (2004). Improving educational services for students with TBI through statewide consulting teams. *Neurorehabilitation, 19(3)*, 219-231.

I hope my "101 Tips" will help other TBI survivors in their quest for lives filled with hope and meaning. Good luck! Kelly B. Darmofal

Kelly Bouldin Darmofal's speech for CareNet (May 2015)

I am a 23-year survivor of **severe traumatic brain injury - TBI.** For anyone here *not yet* familiar with the acronym TBI... I hope today you leave here as familiar with it as you are with BMW... PhD...and PMS!! I've learned over time that what I say isn't as important as HOW FAST I SAY IT, so bear with me...

I'll begin by telling you what happened to me 23 years ago when I was barely fifteen and a freshman in high school. My parents wouldn't let me ride in cars with new 16 year old drivers. However, after cheering for my first JV football game, they finally let me go a few blocks from my home to a Burger King... And my mom *did* strap me into a safety belt before the 18 yr old friend took me for food! I *never* made it home!!

I'm told that a backseat passenger was yelling, and the driver *did not* turn when the road curved. We hit a telephone pole and I was knocked unconscious on the dashboard. Weeks later, following deep coma, I woke up—not knowing where I was—or what had happened. I could not speak... or walk... or even remember my whole name. I suffered a severe closed head injury... a severe TBI. I suffered damage to my right frontal lobe, the left occipital lobe, and brain stem.

I didn't dream in deep coma. I didn't see any angels or white lights... but I do recall waking and feeling terribly confused. *Where was I? Why couldn't I talk? When could I get out of this strange place?* Finally someone put a pencil in my hand...

The first sentence I wrote after my traumatic brain injury was – I'M LOST IN MY MIND! I simply didn't know what was happening, and no matter how many times my mom told me about my wreck, I quickly forgot it. I suffered retrograde and antegrade amnesia... or long and short-term memory loss. Today I still have memory issues, and also receptive and expressive aphasia, or the inability to speak rapidly and clearly at times... but I've come a very long way since 1992.

When I first began to talk in the hospital, it was on the *telephone*. Yes, I was a teenager! One night I called 911 and said 'TAKE ME HOME.'

Where are you, said the dispatcher. "I DON'T KNOW... BUT I WANT TO GO HOME!!"

In November 2014, Modern History Press published my memoir *Lost In My Mind: Recovering From Traumatic Brain Injury*. Today, decades after my personal nightmare, people ask me, "Why write a memoir about a time you can barely remember, and revisit your pain and suffering?" Well, for years

I simply didn't want to remember those horrible days. I wanted to be normal again. However, when I returned to public high school, none of my teachers were trained to work with a TBI survivor. I didn't have a true transition team.

Therefore, in high school most teachers thought I was a total disaster. I limped. I drooled. I forgot where my classes were. I couldn't speak with clarity. I was also legally blind. A TBI can affect the entire body.

Without prior training, most teachers could not accept the fact that, in a year or two, I would be making A's. They just knew what they saw, and it wasn't pretty. My social life was a mess. I didn't forget people's names, but I *did* forget how I emotionally felt about them. I'd forgotten my own personality, and I felt depressed and isolated.

However, my problem was mainly that I DID NOT KNOW WHAT *I DID NOT KNOW!* My untrained teachers could not understand, for instance, why *I took notes in the middle of notebooks.* I needed someone to remind me to read and write from left to right – which is an acquired skill I had forgotten.

I can only imagine what my early teachers thought of me. Both of my hands shook constantly. I cussed on occasion. My questions surprised them.

One day I asked, "Who the hell are Matthew, Mark, Luke and John?" Clearly, teachers could not comprehend that I was *healing*. That I would indeed be able to write eventually. That I would remember the four Gospels. If only they had been prepared to meet someone like me! Yes, each TBI is unique, but teachers must learn that we have basic similarities.

Without this knowledge some were kind, and others were condescending. If I forgot homework, or couldn't read the blackboard, some teachers penalized me ... instead of saying, "Kelly, you'll be better soon... let me help you and copy your assignments!"

The best teachers had natural empathy. For example, my geometry teacher let me number my theorems instead of copying full sentences.

My history teacher allowed me to retake tests at need....certainly some teachers figured out that, in time, I would regain many lost skills.

But school was a culture shock for me. As an A student, I was used to respect and kindness. As a disabled student, I often experienced discouragement. Yes, I was lucky to be there at all. But I was the first classified TBI survivor in my high school... and teachers were afraid to set precedents until they knew more about TBI... and they are still waiting. Teaching programs in 2015 generally ignore the TBI category... which is a mystery to me... because there are millions of TBI survivors in our public schools!

I'll give you examples of my short term memory problems – My teachers had the annoying habit of **postponing tests**.... a horrible thing for the student with TBI who studied all night to remember facts *for maybe 24 hours...* and had to study again and again until the test actually occurred. Despite my IEP, few teachers discovered how little help I really needed—like Xeroxed notes.

Another example: I didn't know clothes had to match, and often combined winter and summer clothing. Some days I put on one white shoe and one black shoe... because dressing well is an acquired skill, a learned skill... and I didn't have it anymore. Therefore, teachers saw me in green socks and hiking boots... the only shoes that would support my weak ankles... they probably assumed my IQ was as weak as my wardrobe skills.

Years later, after rehab and high school, I entered college. I benefited from the excellent counseling recommended at Brenner Children's Hospital. Counseling saved my life...as surely as the doctors at Wake Forest/BMC. But, I was still struggling for lost memories and skills.

In college few teachers were trained to help a student with TBI. Later, in graduate school, the same problems reoccurred. My slower speech often was mistaken for a low intelligence. I decided it was time to write a memoir.

Do you know that TBI is the greatest cause of child death in America? It is also the leading cause of disability in young adults in all industrialized nations. TBI is not a condition for soldiers and athletes <u>alone.</u> Our children are in danger: They fall.

They endure abuse. They suffer TBIs in car crashes —and the public isn't noticing their needs.

Most of you have heard of special education—for example, the blind, deaf, or autistic. Our schools have 14 disability categories under the Individuals with Disabilities Education Act or IDEA.

Of these 14 groups, *students with TBI are healing*. Students with TBI can recover more rapidly with trained assistance... but teachers can also do harm to survivors who only seem irreparably impaired. Those with TBI are at **high risk of suicide**, and those who work with us need information and greater awareness.

I stand here as living proof that TBI survivors can dare to hope for recovery. Yet—today, to my knowledge, there are no *4-year liberal arts colleges* that offer undergraduate courses for teachers concerning TBI. George Washington University has begun a graduate program regarding TBI...and I just received some wonderful news: I will be instructing an experimental course for undergraduates at Salem College in 2016; the working title is: "TBI: An Overview For Educators." I hope some of you will help me!

In the last decade I've worked with special needs children – after obtaining a masters degree. Most days I have no problems as a teacher. However, I do need to keep a careful calendar.

One day in the hallway of school, a colleague alerted me to a schedule change... I quickly wrote this change on my arm. My desk was far away. A 2nd grader named Noah, asked me, "Ms. Darmofal, why did you write on your arm??"

"I need to remember this meeting, Noah," I answered, "and I may forget it...my memory isn't too great." He responded:

"Ms. Darmofal, I think I'd rather just stay clean!"

Well, so would I, I said to Noah. I'm just doing the best I can with the cards I've been dealt.... which is true of most people everywhere!

For precious students like Noah, who are at great risk of TBI, I did complete my story for publication. My story was endorsed by the President/CEO of the BIAA (Brain Injury Association of America).

I'd like to read you something Susan Connors wrote with colleagues just months ago:

"TBI is not an orphan disease affecting only 25,000 children... currently up to seven million U.S. school children (age 5-15) may have experienced a brain injury...". Today research proves TBI is not a "low incidence" category, as once believed. TBI is a HIGH INCIDENCE condition, and schools must attend.

In 2005 I wrote an article for *English Journal* titled "TBI: Our Teachers are Not Prepared" – this fact must change!!! Our hospitals and non-profits cannot do the work alone. I believe in **diagnostic teaching.** We *know TBI survivors are under-*

identified. Teachers can help identify them if they know what to look for.

Before I stop, I perhaps should express again the most important message in my personal story, which is:

When someone suffers a TBI, it's essential to HOPE, AND KEEP RIGHT ON HOPING FOR RECOVERY! Many of you know someone who has had a concussion…actually ¾ of all TBIs are mild concussions…but these can lead to symptoms like memory loss and confusion…even personality changes. While each TBI is different, victims and their caretakers need to know that life can improve… the symptoms may be combated with effort. For students with TBI, teachers must help survivors regain their lost abilities. Personally, I never gave up hoping for a full recovery. <u>Hope</u> is my message. Never give up the fight!

As Emily Dickenson wrote:

> "Hope" is the thing with feathers –
> That perches in the soul—
> And sings the tune without the words—
> And never stops——at all.

I'll close with a Bible verse sent to me by my guardian angel Britt Armfield, who died in a car crash in 1993 and still speaks to me:

> "I consider that our present sufferings are not worth comparing with the glory that will be revealed in us." – ROMANS 8:18

About the Author

Kelly Bouldin Darmofal is a teacher, author, wife, motivational speaker and mother to a perfect, three year old son named Alex. Because she suffered a severe closed head injury (traumatic brain injury) in 1992, and endured a lengthy convalescence, Kelly now advocates for the survivors of TBI in America—especially students. She has written a memoir, spanning three decades of recovery entitled, *Lost in My Mind: Recovering from Traumatic Brain Injury (TBI)*. Kelly's journey is unique in its focus on education (or lack thereof) for TBI survivors in America.

Kelly's memoir was published by Modern History Press (MHP) in October, 2014, and has been endorsed by Susan Connors, the President and CEO of the Brain Injury Association of America (BIAA). In January of 2016, Kelly will instruct such a course entitled, "TBI—An Overview for Educators" (working title) at Salem College in North Carolina. This innovative class will be the first of its kind offered in a four year, undergraduate liberal arts college or university in America. With millions of students returning to the classroom annually with traumatic brain injuries, such a course is a necessity.

Prior to publishing *Lost in My Mind: Recovering from TBI*, Kelly had written an article, "Our Teachers Are Not Prepared" (English Journal, 2005), which won a prestigious Edwin M. Hopkins Award from the NCTE, or National Council of Teachers of English. Kelly obtained her Masters in Special Education from Salem College in Winston-Salem, North Carolina, and has taught special education at Forsyth Country Day School and Summit School in Winston-Salem.

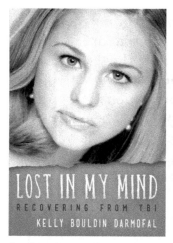

Lost in My Mind is a stunning memoir describing Kelly Bouldin Darmofal's journey from adolescent girl to special education teacher, wife and mother — despite severe Traumatic Brain Injury (TBI). Spanning three decades, Kelly's journey is unique in its focus on TBI education in America (or lack thereof). Kelly also abridges her mother's journals to describe forgotten experiences. She continues the narrative in her own humorous, poetic voice, describing a victim's relentless search for success, love, and acceptance — while combating bureaucratic red tape, aphasia, bilateral hand impairment, and loss of memory.

"This peek into the real-life trials and triumphs of a young woman, who survives a horrific car crash and struggles to regain academic excellence and meaningful social relationships, is a worthwhile read for anyone who needs information, inspiration, or escape from the isolation so common after traumatic brain injury."

Susan H. Connors, President/CEO,
Brain Injury Association of America

ISBN 978-1-61599-244-7

NOTES

CPSIA information can be obtained
at www.ICGtesting.com
Printed in the USA
BVHW091048180421
605249BV00002B/36

9 781615 994335